CONTENTS

Weight Loss with Small Habit Changes

The KISS Method: Achieve weight loss without resorting to extreme diets.

Janet M. Edwards

Wacky Publications

DEDICATION

To my parents, whose unwavering love and faith in me have been my greatest strength. And to my cousin Marie for her inspiration to start writing.

INTRODUCTION

Overview of Mini Habits

The mini habits approach is about making tiny, easy changes to build lasting habits. Instead of setting big, hard-to-reach goals, mini habits focus on small steps, like reading one page of a book or doing one push-up a day. These goals are so small that they're easy to do, helping you start without feeling overwhelmed. As you repeat these tiny actions, they start to feel natural, often leading you to do even more. Mini habits build consistency and don't rely on willpower or motivation. Over time, these small actions add up, creating big and lasting changes in your life.

Why Traditional Diets Fail

Traditional diets often fail because they're too extreme and hard to stick with. Many diets ask for a big overhaul of your eating habits right away, cutting out favorite foods or reducing calories too much. This can make you feel deprived, frustrated, or even tired, making it hard to keep going. When diets are too strict, they rely on willpower, which can run out over time, especially when life gets stressful.

Another problem with traditional diets is that they're usually short-term, focused on quick results rather than lasting change. Once the diet ends, many people go back to old eating habits and regain the weight they lost.

Mini habits take a different approach by focusing on small, easy-to-maintain changes. Instead of aiming for huge, immediate results, mini habits encourage tiny steps, like adding one healthy food or drinking more water. These small changes are easy to keep up and can gradually build into bigger, healthier routines. By focusing on what feels like little habits it helps create lasting habits without the stress or frustration of traditional diets.

CHAPTER ONE –
THE BEGINNING

I'm not a doctor, nurse, or nutritionist, just a regular person who has been trying to lose weight for years with some success. I used to weigh 250 pounds, and nothing seemed to work no matter what diet I tried. Then I met my husband, and without any special diet, I lost 20 pounds by just going with the flow and enjoying life.

Later, I got pregnant with my first child. During the pregnancy, I got very sick and ended up losing 60 pounds. Thankfully, my child turned out healthy and wonderful. When I had my second child, I didn't get sick, but he was a difficult baby and was later diagnosed with autism. Around that time, we also moved, and I gained back the 60 pounds I had lost.

For years, my weight stayed the same until about five years ago when I took a 7-week class on eating "Whole Foods, Plant-Based" diet. I lost 20 pounds during the class but got sick again. I recovered, but my health challenges didn't stop there. Years ago, I was injured in an accident and have been in a wheelchair ever since. This causes painful sores that sometimes require plastic surgery to fix, making exercise very hard for me.

The Whole Foods diet worked for a while, but I got bored, like I do with most diets, so I stopped. Luckily, I didn't gain weight back. Two years ago, I had a mild heart attack

—so mild I drove myself to the hospital, which was only a mile away. That's when I learned I had high cholesterol and finally started taking statins after refusing them for a long time. I lost another 25 pounds but started dealing with severe constipation, which has been very painful. At one point, I didn't go for 16 days straight. It's better now, but still a struggle.

Even with all these challenges, my weight is down, and I've found ways to lose more without dieting. Over the past three months, I've lost another 10 pounds, and I feel more empowered than ever. I want to share what's worked for me so others can lose weight without going on restrictive diets.

To Weigh or not to Weigh

Some experts recommend weighing yourself daily, but I disagree. Daily weigh-ins can be discouraging because you might not see much change, and weight can fluctuate for reasons like drinking extra water. Here's what I suggest:

1. Use the same scale and weigh yourself once a week.

2. Weigh yourself in the morning after first using the bathroom.

3. Wear the same clothes or nothing at all for consistency.

This gives you the most accurate results. Remember, slow and steady weight loss is more sustainable. Even losing one pound a week adds up to 50 pounds in a year—an amazing achievement if you keep it off!

Get a Checkup

Before starting this journey, I recommend visiting your doctor for a checkup. There could be underlying health issues affecting your weight, such as high cholesterol, diabetes, Celiac disease, or other conditions. For example, taking medication for high cholesterol has helped me, and my aunt lost a significant amount of weight after discovering she had Celiac disease, a gluten allergy. Understanding any hidden health factors can make a big difference in your ability to lose weight or prevent weight gain.

CHAPTER TWO

- HEALTHY EATING

Where do I start

Many times, I've thought, *"Can someone just tell me what to do? Just tell me what to eat!"* I understand that feeling, and I'm here to help. I've been on this journey many times, and I'm finally making progress. The key is to take it one step at a time, so it doesn't feel overwhelming.

I call my approach the **KISS Method**—*Keep It Simple, Silly*. After searching for answers my whole life, I've realized it's about acting and listening to my body to find the most natural path forward. For me, that means eating plenty of vegetables and fruits, still enjoying some meat, and limiting starches.

But before diving into food choices, it's important to start with habits that can naturally slow down your eating—without changing your diet at all.

Hydration Habit

Building a hydration habit is one of the simplest ways to improve your health. A great way to start is by drinking one glass of water before meals or first thing in the morning. This small step is easy to add to your daily routine and can have a big impact over time.

Drinking water in the morning helps wake up your body and boosts your energy after hours without fluids. Before meals, a glass of water can help with digestion and even prevent overeating by making you feel fuller.

This habit is simple because it doesn't require much effort or planning. Experts recommend drinking eight glasses of water a day, not including other beverages. I've tried this, and if you drink all eight glasses in one day, you may find yourself spending a lot of time in the bathroom the next day. Instead, try adding an extra glass of water each day or every few days to ease into the habit.

You can keep a glass by your bed or a water bottle in the kitchen as a reminder. Over time, this small step can grow into a steady routine of drinking more water throughout the day. Staying hydrated is essential for healthy skin, energy, and focus, and starting with just one glass is an easy way to begin.

One Veggie Per Meal

Adding more vegetables to your diet can be simple if you start small. Begin by adding just one serving of vegetables to one meal each day. This could be broccoli with dinner, a handful of spinach in your sandwich, or some carrot sticks as a snack. Once this becomes a habit, you can add a second serving to another meal.

Vegetables are full of nutrients your body needs, like vitamins, minerals, and fiber. Eating them regularly can improve digestion, boost your energy, and help you feel fuller for longer. Starting with one serving makes it easy and doesn't feel overwhelming.

To make it even simpler, try frozen or pre-cut veggies for

quick prep. You can also mix them into foods you already enjoy, like soups, pasta, or smoothies. Over time, adding more vegetables will feel natural, and you'll be on your way to a healthier diet without making big, stressful changes.

Mindful Eating Mini Steps

Mindful eating means paying attention to your food and how you eat. It can help you enjoy meals more and avoid overeating. While experts often suggest eating without distractions, I prefer having something to do during meals, like watching the news or, even better, eating with others. Sharing a meal with family or friends can make it more enjoyable and meaningful. However, it's important to stay aware of how much you're eating.

My son, for example, often rushes through his dinner, finishing in minutes, which can lead to overeating or not feeling satisfied. To avoid mindless eating, serve yourself a smaller portion rather than eating straight from a bag or container. This helps you keep track of how much you're consuming.

The "Pause Before Eating" Habit

Pausing before eating habits is a simple way to slow down and enjoy your food. Before taking a bite, pause for a moment. You can take a deep breath, have a sip of water, or just set your fork down. This small habit helps you eat more mindfully and avoid rushing through your meals.

Eating too fast can lead to overeating because it takes time for your brain to realize you're full. By pausing, you give your body a chance to catch up and notice when it's satisfied. This can help you enjoy your meals more and avoid feeling too full afterward.

Start with one meal a day. Take a deep breath before your first bite and try to pause between bites as well. Over time, this habit can become natural. It's an easy way to build mindfulness into your eating, making meals more enjoyable while helping you feel more in control of how much you eat.

The Snack Habit

Snacking can be a healthy part of your day if you do it the right way. Controlling your snack habit starts with planning and being aware of what and how much you eat. Instead of grabbing chips or candy, choose healthier options like fruits, nuts, or yogurt. Always serve your snacks in a small bowl or plate instead of eating straight from the bag or box. This helps you keep track of how much you're eating.

With family and friends, you can make snacking a positive habit by setting good examples. Offer healthy snacks when hosting or share your healthy choices with others. Try making snacks a fun and social activity, like preparing veggie sticks with dips or making fruit skewers together.

It's also helpful to set limits on when and where snacking happens, like avoiding snacks in front of the TV. This helps everyone stay aware of their eating. Snacking doesn't have to be a problem if you keep portions small, make smart food choices, and focus on enjoying the food and company. Small changes can make snacking healthier for you and the people around you.

Another helpful tip is "out of sight, out of mind." If

unhealthy snacks like chips are tucked away in a cupboard, you're less likely to reach for them. For example, when I took my granddaughter out for Halloween, we filled a small bucket with candy. That night, I had one piece and made sure the rest was put away. Even though I know exactly where it is, I haven't had a single piece since then.

The same strategy works for other tempting treats that someone in the house might buy or make. By keeping them stored and out of easy reach, you can avoid mindless snacking and stay in control. This simple habit helps create a healthier environment and makes it easier to stick to better choices.

Portion Control

Portion control is a simple way to eat healthier without feeling like you're giving up your favorite foods. One easy trick is to use smaller plates. A smaller plate makes your portions look larger, which can help your brain feel satisfied with less food. For example, I started using salad plates for dinner instead of regular plates, and it worked! My meals felt just as filling, but I ate less without even trying.

Another helpful tip is to start with half portions. Serve yourself a regular portion, then divide it in half, placing one half on a separate plate to save for tomorrow. When dining out, I ask for half of my meal to be packed up right away, so I'm not tempted to overeat. At home, I dish up smaller amounts and only take more if I'm still genuinely hungry. Most of the time, I find that the smaller portion is just enough.

Did you know that using a small spoon or fork can help you eat more slowly? I decided to test this with my family during a soup dinner. My husband chose a big spoon, while the rest of us used smaller ones. For context, we're all a bit overweight, though not obese.

It's easy to overeat when portions aren't controlled, but small steps like these can make a big difference. By focusing on portion sizes, you can enjoy your meals while staying mindful of how much you're eating.

CHAPTER THREE – OTHER HEALTH ISSUES

Constipation vs. Diarrhea

Maintaining regular bowel movements is key to good health. You should aim to go once each day at a consistent time. Irregularity can cause discomfort, such as constipation or diarrhea. This can harm your well-being.

Managing Constipation

If you don't go often enough, you may experience pain and constipation. I have severe constipation. I tried various over-the-counter remedies, with mixed results. Over time, I've found that certain foods have been particularly helpful. However, moderation is crucial. Overindulging in these foods may cause the opposite problem.

The best foods for easing constipation are fruits. I love raisins and prunes. Other fruits, like plums, watermelon, and apples, can help too. (Check out my recipe for dried apples below!) Teas and milk have helped me, but my go-to is popcorn made with oil or from a microwave pack.

My mother used to tell me about how, in the 1930s and 1940s, castor oil served as a daily remedy for constipation. I prefer using food instead it's much more enjoyable!

Diarrhea

Dealing with diarrhea is a troublesome condition. It can be

harmful if it lasts too long. Staying hydrated is essential when dealing with diarrhea. The recommended diet is the BRAT method: Bananas, Rice, Applesauce, and Toast. These foods can help stabilize digestion.

If diarrhea lasts more than a day or two, see a doctor. Prolonged diarrhea can be very harmful to your health.

Alcohol

The original Weight Watchers Diet discouraged alcohol. Some experts say a small amount of wine may be healthy. The latest guidelines recommend that women limit themselves to one drink a day and men to two.

These recommendations apply regardless of whether you're dieting. If you're trying to lose weight, avoid alcohol. It adds calories and slows your progress.

Smoking

Researchers estimate that smoking one cigarette shortens life by 11 minutes. Long-term smokers lose about 10 years of life expectancy compared to non-smokers. However, the impact varies. It depends on health and smoking frequency.

The good news is that quitting smoking has immediate and long-term health benefits. The earlier you quit, the quicker your body recovers. It's not only your lungs. Smoking also harms your heart and blood vessels.

If you want to quit, check online resources for effective strategies. For example, nicotine gum has helped some. But it can cause dependency if not used as directed. Keep in mind that alternatives like vaping or cigars are no safer than cigarettes.

Take the step to quit today—your body will thank you.

Dried Apple Rings

What You'll Need:

- Apples (e.g., Fuji or another firm variety)
- Lemon juice (fresh or bottled)
- Apple peeler (preferably an old-fashioned countertop model)
- Cinnamon or sugar (optional, for flavor)
- Dehydrator

Step 1: Choose Your Apples

Select a firm apple variety for the best results. We use homegrown Fuji apples, which are partly green and red when ripe. While we've also tried Red Delicious, they don't turn out well for drying. Feel free to experiment with other varieties to find your favorite.

Step 2: Prepare the Apples

Using an apple peeler that cores and slices as it peels will save a lot of time, especially if you're processing a large quantity. Old-fashioned countertop peelers work best. If you don't have one, you can peel, core, and slice the apples by hand, but it will take longer.

Once peeled and cored, your apples should resemble curly fries. A single cut will give you multiple slices that are uniform and ideal for drying.

Step 3: Prevent Browning

Place the apple slices into a bowl of lemon juice to keep them from browning. You can use freshly squeezed lemons or bottled lemon juice. Let the slices soak for a few minutes, then shake off any excess juice.

Step 4: Arrange on Dehydrator Trays
Lay the slices in a single layer on the dehydrator trays. You can add flavors like cinnamon. Follow the instructions specific to your dehydrator model. Ensure the machine is in a well-ventilated area to prevent overheating.

Step 5: Dry the Apples
Set the dehydrator to the recommended temperature and dry the apples for 6 to 12 hours. Check the apples periodically, and once they feel dry and leathery with no visible moisture, they are ready. The exact time may vary depending on your dehydrator and how crispy or chewy you prefer the apples.

Step 6: Store the Dried Apples
Once the apples are fully dried and cooled, store them in an airtight container or plastic bag with a desiccant packet to keep them fresh. Properly stored, they can last up to a year and still taste freshly picked.

A Few Tips:

- This process uses only apples and lemon juice—no added sugar, salt, or preservatives. But you can add flavors like cinnamon.

- Be cautious not to eat too many dried apples at once; they can cause digestive issues, as my husband's co-workers discovered after snacking on them all day!

Store-bought dried apples are convenient but often contain added chemicals and calories. Homemade dried apple rings are a healthier, tastier alternative that's well worth the time and effort.

Drying Apples using an Oven

Ingredients

Apples (any variety you like)

Lemon juice (to prevent browning)

Cinnamon or sugar (optional, for flavor)

Instructions

1. Preheat your oven to 200°F (93°C) or use a food dehydrator if you have one.

2. Prepare the Apples - Wash and core the apples. Slice them into thin, even rings or wedges (about 1/8-inch thick) for uniform drying.

3. Prevent Browning - Soak the apple slices in at least 1 tablespoon of lemon juice for about 5 minutes. Drain and shake dry.

4. Add Flavor (Optional) - Sprinkle the apple slices with cinnamon, sugar, or a combination of both for added flavor.

5. Arrange on Baking Sheet - Place the apple slices on a baking sheet lined with parchment paper. Make sure they're in a single layer without overlapping.

6. Dry the Apples - Bake in the oven for 2-3 hours, flipping the slices halfway through. For chewier apples, bake for less time; for crispier apples, bake longer.

7. Cool and Store - Let the dried apples cool completely before storing them in an airtight container. Properly stored, they can last for

months.

Enjoy your homemade dried apples as a healthy snack or a delicious topping for cereals and salads!

CHAPTER FOUR - SOME
SPECIFIC FOODS CHOICES

I remember when Oprah Winfrey and Dr. Phil did a special on weight loss TV program and book, and it didn't resonate with me because it didn't address *what* to eat. In this section, I'll share some tips on how to plan meals that include better food choices. Ultimately, though, it's up to you to decide what foods work for you. If you don't choose food, you enjoy and are willing to eat it , your plan won't stick. Making lasting changes to lose weight or improve your health often requires adjusting your lifestyle.

I've tried a couple of weight-loss programs that provided pre-packaged meals. While I did lose weight, it was mostly because I didn't enjoy the food and ended up eating less.

I do talk about calories in my discussions, but I don't count calories or points regularly. Instead, I use them as a general guide to understand how much I'm consuming. For example, if you go to a fast-food restaurant, you might ask yourself: *Do I really want to spend most of my daily 2,000-calorie average on a double or triple burger, or would a single burger be enough?*

The number of calories you need each day depends on many factors, like your activity level and health, so it's important to do your own research to figure out what works best for you. Work on one meal at a time, breakfast then lunch and finally dinner. This way you do not get stressed with so many changes.

Breakfast

Start by choosing foods that will satisfy your hunger and give you good nutrition. It's a good idea to plan a few different options so you don't get bored. Here are some simple ideas:

1. **Oatmeal with Fruit**
   Add fruits like strawberries, raspberries, blueberries, bananas, or whatever you like. You can mix a few together or keep it simple. Fresh fruit is best, but if it's not in season or too expensive, try frozen or dried. To add flavor, sprinkle in cinnamon or a tiny bit of maple syrup.

2. **Yogurt**
   Pick your favorite yogurt—any flavor or style, like Greek yogurt. Just check the label for added sugar if you're watching that. Yogurt is great for digestion because it has probiotics. For women, especially during or after menopause, it can help prevent certain infections. You can eat it plain or mix it into your oatmeal. Try to have yogurt at least once a week.

3. **Veggie Omelet**
   Occasionally, make an omelet with veggies like mushrooms, onions, bell peppers, or anything else you enjoy. Add a small amount of cheese for flavor. It's a filling breakfast that might even make you skip lunch—but don't do that every day!

4. **Make-Ahead Tortilla Wrap**
   Use leftovers, like an omelet or other favorite

fillings, and wrap them in a tortilla. This is great for busy mornings when you need something ready to grab and go.

The key is to pick options you'll actually eat. If you don't like it, the plan won't work. Having a plan also helps you avoid unhealthy choices, like grabbing a donut. Prepare your breakfast the night before so you can stay on track and still make it to work on time.

Lunch

After you get breakfast sorted, move on to lunch. Here are two simple ideas:

1. **Salads**

   My go-to lunch is salad, but I keep it simple. I buy a mixed greens salad bag that usually has a small amount of bacon, dressing, and other extras. I divide it into three portions for three meals. To make it better, I add a little cheese and sometimes extra veggies like tomatoes.

Some of the extras in these salad kits, like taco strips or sunflower seeds, are high in starch or calories, so I toss them out.

Be careful with single-serving salads you can buy at the store or when you go to a restaurant. These often have lots of ham, chicken, cheese, and dressing—making them more like two meals in one. If you have one of these, try saving some of the meat or cheese for another meal. Portion control is key!

2. **Wraps**

   A good cold wrap can also be a great lunch.

Look for wraps loaded with greens like lettuce or spinach and add other veggies too. I use a small amount of mayo, mustard, or ketchup to keep it from being dry. Keep in mind, wraps have about the same calories as sandwiches, so stick to one wrap and pair it with a piece of fruit, like an apple, to round out the meal.

These ideas focus on balanced portions and variety. Once you've got lunch working for you, you can move on to planning your dinner!

Dinner

Dinner can be a bit trickier than breakfast or lunch because we often must think about feeding the whole family. Here's a simple way to plan your plate:

- **Divide your plate into 4 parts:**
    1. **First quarter:** Choose a small portion of meat (2–3 ounces for women, 3–4 ounces for men).

    2. **Second quarter:** Add a small portion of starch, like bread, rice, or pasta.

    3. **Last half:** Fill it with vegetables—these can be warm or cold, and you can mix them up.

This method helps you enjoy a balanced meal while staying on track with weight loss goals.

Three Ways to Enjoy Your Meal:

1. Eat the same meal as your family but stick to smaller portions.

2. Follow the "quarter plate" method described

above with small portions.

3. Skip the meat and focus on fruits and vegetables—since these are low in calories, you can eat a bit more.

Dessert

Desserts don't have to be heavy. Try making fruit the main treat:

- **Simple options:** Strawberries with a bit of milk and sugar, fresh apples (plain or cooked), or seasonal fruits like watermelon or peaches.

- **Small indulgences:** If you have cake or pie, enjoy it in small portions. For example, if you buy a single-serve cake cut it into four pieces to share with the rest of the family.

The key is not to deny your cravings but enjoy them in moderation. This way, you're less likely to overeat later.

Cooking Tips

- Use **canola oil** or **extra virgin olive oil (EVOO)** for cooking. Both have the same fat and calorie content, but canola oil is cheaper and has a milder taste.

- For a lighter option, cook with **water or stock** (like chicken stock). Add a teaspoon of butter at the end for extra flavor.

Add Flavor with Spices

Spice up your meals with garlic, basil, oregano, or other seasonings. Condiments like mustard, ketchup, or hot sauce are also great. Fun fact: hot sauces might help you eat slower, which can make it easier to eat less.

CHAPTER FIVE –
MOVEMENT OR EXERCISE

One-Minute Workouts

Starting a workout routine can feel overwhelming, but one-minute workouts make it simple. Just start with one minute of movement—stretching, a quick walk, or even a few jumping jacks. If a certain exercise feels too hard, don't worry! There's often an easier way to do it.

For example, instead of traditional pushups on the floor, try "wall pushups." Stand facing a wall, place your hands on it, and use your arms to push your body away from the wall. It's a great alternative that works for many people, including those with limited mobility.

There are many modified exercises designed to be accessible for people with disabilities or different fitness levels. These options make it possible for everyone to get moving and stay active in a way that works best for their body.

Why does this work? One minute is short enough to fit into even the busiest day. It helps you build the habit of moving your body regularly without stress. Over time, these small efforts can grow into longer sessions as you feel more comfortable and motivated.

For example, stretch your arms and legs during a TV break or take a quick walk around your room. These tiny steps add up and can improve your energy, mood, and overall health.

The key is consistency, not intensity. Starting small makes it easier to stick with your goal of staying active. So, don't wait—give it a try today! One minute is all it takes to start a positive change.

How much is enough, a daily amount of consent movement of 5 to 10 minutes is good. The goal is not to run a marathon but consistency. I have heard that 7,000 steps a day is a good amount but do what works for you. You can track steps using a watch device or a pedometer. It is a device designed to count the number of steps a person takes. It typically works by detecting motion or vibrations caused by walking or running. Pedometers are commonly used to track physical activity and encourage movement, helping users monitor their fitness levels. Remember every journey starts with 1 step, don't worry that you are not getting enough, do some and build up to a good number for yourself.

Others mini exercises that add up

- Taking the Stairs: Simple swaps for daily activity, like choosing stairs over elevators.

- Stand and Stretch: Adding a few standing or stretching breaks throughout the day to keep active.

- Incremental Exercise Builds: Gradually increasing workout time or intensity based on success with smaller activities.

Online Resources for Exercise

Getting active is easier with online resources. You can

find pre-recorded exercises and group sessions to fit your needs and schedule.

Pre-recorded exercise videos are great because you can watch and follow them anytime, anywhere. There are videos for all fitness levels, from beginners to advanced. You can choose from yoga, stretching, dancing, strength training, and more. With so many options, it's easy to find something you enjoy.

Group sessions online offer another way to stay active. These are live classes where you can join others in real-time. It's a fun way to feel connected, even from home. Many group sessions have instructors who guide you through the workout and keep you motivated.

Whether you want to work out alone or feel part of a group, online resources make exercise convenient and flexible. All you need is a device with internet access, and you're ready to go. With so many choices available, there's something for everyone to stay active and healthy. Try looking on You Tube or for a local fitness group that you can participate with and not leave your home.

The Buddy System: Stay Active Together

Exercising with a friend or co-worker is a great way to stay consistent with your workouts and it works for meals as well. This is called the "buddy system," and it works because having someone by your side makes exercise more fun and less of a chore.

A workout buddy can motivate you to show up, even on days when you don't feel like it. You can cheer each other on and set goals together. Whether it's a walk during lunch breaks, a gym session, or a quick online workout, doing it together keeps you both on track.

The buddy system also makes exercise feel less lonely. You can chat, laugh, and even challenge each other to try new activities. Plus, it's easier to stick to a routine when someone else is counting on you.

Find a friend or co-worker with similar fitness goals and schedule regular times to exercise. Even a short session together can boost your mood and energy. With a buddy, staying active becomes something you look forward to, not just another task.

Your best workout buddy might just be your spouse or partner. They're often around in the evenings for a short walk or available on weekends for adventures that combine exercise and sightseeing. Plus, exercising together can start with something as simple, and enjoyable, as a kiss!

Find a Hobby: The Benefits of Having a Hobby

1. **Keeps your hands busy**: When your hands are doing something, they're not grabbing snacks from the kitchen.

2. **Relieves stress**: A creative hobby can help you relax while giving your brain something new to work on.

3. **Gets you out of the house**: Hobbies can lead to meeting new people in groups, sharing experiences, and spending less time thinking

about food.

4. **Might lead to something more**: Some hobbies, like playing in a band or crafting, could even grow into a career.

Simple hobbies include knitting, puzzles, or anything else you enjoy. If you can't find a hobby, try volunteering—it's a great way to stay busy and help others.

CHAPTER SIX - BETTER SLEEP

Bedtime Routine Basics

Creating a simple bedtime routine can make a big difference in how well you sleep. Start by introducing one relaxing activity before bed. This could be reading a book, listening to music, stretching with yoga, short meditations or even practicing deep breathing exercises. These calming activities signal to your body that it's time to wind down. This will move your focus away from daily stress, while gentle stretches can release tension built up during the day.

Consistency is key, try to do the same activity every night to train your mind and body to recognize your bedtime cues. Keep the atmosphere calm by dimming the lights and reducing screen time by at least an hour before bed. Slip into soft, soothing pajamas that keep you comfortable at the perfect temperature. By making one simple adjustment to your nightly routine, you'll enjoy better sleep and more restful nights.

Consistent Sleep Times

Maintaining a consistent sleep schedule can improve your overall sleep quality. Try setting a regular bedtime and wake-up time, keeping them within a 30-minute range each day, even on weekends.

This consistency helps regulate your body's internal clock, making it easier to fall asleep and wake up feeling refreshed. Over time, your body will naturally adjust to this routine, reducing the need for alarms or struggling to get out of bed. To make this work, choose times that fit your lifestyle and allow for enough sleep—ideally 7–9 hours for most adults. Avoid drastic changes, as they can disrupt your rhythm and leave you feeling groggy. Maintaining a consistent sleep schedule is a straightforward yet impactful way to improve sleep quality and overall health. This practice benefits everyone, from infants to teenagers. They even have a name for it, called maintaining your circadian rhythm.

Technology Timeout

Taking a break from screens before bed can help you sleep better. Try turning off your phone, tablet, or TV at least 15 minutes before bedtime. The blue light from screens can confuse your brain and make it harder to relax and fall asleep. By giving yourself a technology timeout, you allow your mind and body to wind down naturally.

Use this time for something calming instead. You could read a book, do light stretches, or simply enjoy some quiet moments. These activities help your brain recognize it's time to get ready for sleep. Start small, just 15 minutes without screens before bed and see how it feels. Over time, you may notice that you fall asleep faster and wake up feeling more rested.

Make your Bedroom like a Bat Cave

Turning your bedroom into a peaceful "bat cave" can help you sleep better. It's all about keeping your room dark, quiet, and cozy.

Start by blocking out light. Use blackout curtains or blinds to keep outside light from sneaking in. If that's not possible, try a sleep mask. Inside your room, keep lights dim or off, and avoid glowing clocks or electronics.

If you need to read a clock at night, find one with adjustable brightness. I found a great clock that lets me dim it to different levels, which is helpful. Another option is to point your clock face down so the light doesn't shine on you. This makes it easy to move and check when needed without disturbing your sleep.

Next, reduce noise. Use earplugs if you live in a noisy area or turn on a white noise machine or fan to block out distracting sounds. Make your room feel calm and comfortable. Keep it cool, around 60–67°F, and use soft, cozy bedding. These small changes can turn your room into the perfect place for deep, restful sleep.

CHAPTER SEVEN –
SOLUTIONS TO FOOD TRIGGERS

Planning and Family obligations.

The hardest question for many moms is, "What's for dinner?" Planning meals ahead of time can save money and help you eat healthier. When you know what's for dinner each night, you're less likely to spend on last-minute takeout or grab unnecessary items at the store.

Start by making a weekly meal plan. Write down what you'll cook each day and create a shopping list. To save even more time, organize your list by the aisles of your store. I've made a spreadsheet of my store's layout that I can quickly reprint or use on my phone. The faster you shop, the fewer unnecessary items you'll grab, and the less often you'll need to go to the store—one or two trips a week should be enough.

Meal planning doesn't have to be complicated. Pick easy recipes or prep ingredients ahead of time. Some families go a step further by cooking in bulk a couple of times a week and freezing meals. Later, they simply heat up a prepared meal and enjoy.

With just a little planning, you'll save money, eat better, and feel more organized during the week.

Recognizing Triggers

Make a list of the things that make you want to eat when you're not hungry. Pick one at a time and think of ways to handle it. Ask yourself, *What can I do instead?* Try replacing eating with small habits, like going for a short walk, to help deal with your feelings.

Examples of some of my bad habits and solutions

1. **Eating late at night**:
   - Set a time to stop eating, like 8 p.m.
   - Brush your teeth after dinner and remind yourself, *I don't eat after brushing.*
   - Clean the kitchen, turn off the lights, and only go in for only water or no-calorie drinks.

2. **Buying junk food**:
   - Stop buying chips, candy, and sweets and bringing them home. It's easier to say no at the store than to resist them at home all week.
   - Shop with someone else. For example, I shop with my husband, and I'm less likely to buy unhealthy snacks when he is with me.

Mini Habits for Progress

1. **Track small habits**: Use a notebook or an app to track your progress. Even if you don't write everything down, notice your bad habits, then you can work on replacing them with good habits.

2. **Think "1% better"**: Don't aim for perfection—just try to make small improvements. For example, if you want to stop eating after dinner, start by eating a little less of those foods each night. Progress adds up over time.

3. **Be patient**: Weight loss is a journey, not a race. Focus on building habits that improve your life in the long run.

CONCLUSION

Small Changes, Big Results

There's no magic pill for weight loss, nor is there a perfect diet that will solve everything instantly. However, small, consistent habits can create significant change over time. Instead of chasing quick fixes, focus on identifying and addressing the small barriers that hold you back.

You don't need to eat foods you dislike—stick with what works for you. Start with one meal at a time. For example, set up a routine for breakfast that's healthy, quick, and easy, so you don't overeat. Once breakfast becomes second nature, apply the same strategy to lunch and dinner. Gradually eat slightly smaller portions, and you'll find your hunger adjusts, and the pounds will begin to drop.

After establishing a solid food routine, add small amounts of exercise to your day. Don't forget the importance of sleep, it plays a critical role in overall health and weight loss.

The toughest habit of addressing emotional triggers is managing emotional triggers. These triggers, ingrained over years, often drive unhealthy behaviors. Change takes time, so tackle them one by one. As you feel the positive effects of healthy eating, you'll be better equipped to handle these challenges.

Remember: **Keep It Simple, Silly (KISS)**. Celebrate small victories, cherish your loved ones, and embrace a lifestyle that leads to a longer, healthier, and happier life.

REFERENCES

Manaker, L. (2024, October 29). *The 11 Best Yogurts for Weight Loss, According to Dietitians*. Eat this. Retrieved November 14, 2024, from https://www.eatthis.com/best-yogurts-for-weight-loss/

Scott, S. (2015, February 19). *22 Benefits of Having a Hobby or Enjoying a Leisure Activity*. Develop good habits. Retrieved November 24, 2024, from https://www.developgoodhabits.com/benefits-hobby/